WILD HORSE,
Wild Heart

INSPIRING STORIES, PRACTICES, AND REFLECTIONS TO LIBERATE THE HORSE WITHIN.

DINA VARELLAS

Dina Varellas
Contact Information – dvarellasyoga@gmail.com or
dinavarellas.com.

Wild Horse, Wild Heart / Dina Varellas—1st ed.
ISBN 978-0-578-32254-4

*"Blame it or praise it; there is no denying
the wild horse in us."*

VIRGINIA WOOLF

I dedicate this book to my dad, who always told me I should write a book. This one is for you, Pops. Thank you for believing in me and encouraging me to follow my dreams.

To Rachel — my dear friend, sister, and first trainer. Thank you for your generous and patient heart, for welcoming me into the world of horses, holding space, and creating the conditions for healing and transformation.

To Cody — the first horse to steal my heart and awaken me to the mystery and beauty of horses. Thank you for your loyal companionship.

How to Use This Book

In this book, I will share with you my journey and personal stories with Cody and horses. The practices and writing prompts I suggest are designed to help you slow down and tune in, and uncover and discover deeper meaning, joy, and purpose — creating the conditions for a richer life.

The practices and reflections are designed for anyone. Prior experience or knowledge of horses, owning one, or being near a horse is not required. The only prerequisite is a curious and willing heart and mind. If the opportunity arises and wonder piques, I highly recommend spending some time with them. Horses teach us a lot about life and ourselves.

Something about being with a horse offers a powerful invitation to slow down, breathe, become present in our bodies and surroundings, and connect with our hearts. One of the most powerful life lessons that horses offer us is that everything begins with exploring the relationship with ourselves.

This book is an invitation to slow down and rest your mind. You can read in sequential order, chapter by chapter, or you can skip around to the beginning, middle, and end. The book is a tool to support you. There is no right or wrong way to approach the practices and prompts.

I invite you to read with a compassionate, open mind. Kindness gives us the strength to explore and gracefully care for our deepest truths and wounds, to become curious as we explore uncharted territory.

There are blank pages after each chapter for notes and personal reflection. Write what is real and alive inside of you. Trust whatever comes out on the page. All your thoughts and feelings hold truth, power, and value.

Whether you're looking for a source to inspire and uplift, or reflect and nourish, or reacquaint yourself with your natural abilities, I am honored to share my journey with you and to help restore and connect you to your sense of inspiration, courage, passion, faith, infinite capacity, and resilience.

May this book inspire, heal, and evoke the horse within and encourage you to answer the call of your heart and reconnect with the untamed horse within.

Thank you for reading.

Honoring Inspiration

"In out-of-the-way places of the heart,
Where your thoughts never think to wander,
This beginning has been quietly forming,
Waiting until you were ready to emerge."

JOHN O'DONOHUE

For many years I felt a restlessness. It would come and go depending on the seasons and circumstances of my life. But she always returned. She was reliable in that way. A subtle undertone, a persistent ache, was calling me closer to my heart.

My spirit longed for something — adventure, excitement, joy. Something was missing, but I didn't know what. The reoccurring narrative around this idea that I should be doing, venturing, and traveling more repeated within me. These things would satisfy my soul temporarily but never quenched my internal yearning.

Like the familiar hum of a Fleetwood Mac melody, she reminded me that growth and healing would not happen by standing still. I needed to expand and stretch beyond comfort and trust the limitless potential of the unknown and the call in my heart.

It would be years before I recognized the desire for change and had the clarity and courage to answer the call of curiosity. Years of devoted inner work, life's unpredictability, and events aligned forecasting what was to come.

At the onset of the pandemic, my husband and I hiked daily in the open spaces in my hometown of Walnut Creek, CA. Ranches and stables surround the foothills of Mount Diablo and the places we walked and explored. On occasion, we passed a rider on horseback. As I walked past, I could feel the horse's subtle breath kiss my skin, their scent an aphrodisiac — a slight current vibrating my heart.

My relentless curiosity around horses grew. I felt a pull, a deep desire to learn more about these mystical beings. I planted seeds and became aware of the signs. I expressed to my husband my desire to take horseback riding lessons in 2021 — the architecture of how, when, where, and with who yet to be outlined.

In November 2020, Rachel Winner was referred to my Intuitive Writing for Women class. I got to know Rachel intimately as I witnessed vulnerable stories of heartache, perseverance, strength, bravery, beauty, and love. I invited Rachel to continue her healing journey and join me in the winter as I led her and a group of women on a 10-week journey of The Practice®. In exchange, I would spend a few sessions with her practicing equine therapy and learning how to ride and care for a horse at her ranch in Petaluma, CA. It was Rachel's generous and willing heart that would connect me to her lifetime love and knowledge of horses.

I was about to embark on a voyage with no compass or map to refer to, only the call of curiosity and the sweet taste of inspiration.

People come into and leave our lives for reasons sometimes we can't explain or pay attention to. But if we stretch our minds, undefend our hearts, listen, and align with the cues and signs life places in our path, we grow, expand, and expose ourselves to opportunity.

This is a tale of romance between a woman and a horse. A story of the wonder and magic of the Universe, on connection and chasing curiosity, and learning how to rest our minds. And, when we do, how it creates the ability to hear the language of our soul in the many ways it speaks to us through inspiration and intuition, unleashing our infinite potential.

CHAPTER 1

Answering the Call

*"Sometimes the bravest and most important thing
you can do is just show up."*

BRENÉ BROWN

Rachel and I set a date for me to visit her and the horses — December 26. Though weeks away, I already had butterflies in my stomach. The seeds and fruits of my intention earlier in the year were unfolding and aligning in ways I never imagined.

My birthday and holidays were not the usual delights. There was a sense of heaviness, a sadness alongside the joy and celebration.

As the days approached, thoughts of postponing our session entered my mind. I learned the sad and scary news that my dad had contracted COVID-19 while staying in an assisted rehab center. A place he had been residing for a couple of months after an unconscious episode and fall in his one-bedroom assisted living apartment. After months of lockdown and isolation, he was alone again, sick with disease, uncomfortable, and confused. What would happen over the next couple of weeks? Would he survive, a man already with his fair share of illness? It was heartbreaking and challenging to witness and sit in the uncertainty.

The weather, much like my moods, was a dance between scattered rains, gray clouds, and sunshine. Would the rain delay my lesson? Part of me secretly hoped.

Here I was on the edge of my dream, but familiar feelings of discomfort crept in, and the habit of staying home felt too easy. Even if I wanted to be there, showing up to anything new was always highly uncomfortable. It still is because for more than thirty years I considered myself reserved, and going to anything new, especially without having a companion for emotional support, was not typical behavior.

My emotional fatigue and uneasiness started to question my inspiration, the desire to learn how to ride, and the benefits of equine therapy. Was I going to drive to Petaluma the morning after Christmas? It sounded exhausting, beautiful, and intimidating.

My courage and curiosity got the best of me. It was my higher self and the Universe that got me up early and out of the house that morning. A day I would never look back on with regret.

Upon arrival, Rachel showed me around the ranch. She introduced me to Cody, a 23-year-old, seasoned, flea-bitten, gray paint draft horse with soulful amber eyes the color of sweet southern molasses, a light pink muzzle with patches of gray, and a mane and tale the color of creamy vanilla bean. I was immediately attracted to his calm demeanor, and it was decided I would work with him. The introductions continued with Finn, a 10-year-old, flea-bitten, sexy Arabian; Selena, a 4-year-old rescued, Blood Bay Devil's Garden wild mustang with sass and grace; Jimmy, a 5-year old dachshund Chihuahua; and Otis, a nine-year-old pug Chihuahua.

That day I learned horsemanship skills — cleaning hooves,

grooming, and brushing Cody's body, mane, and tail. I practiced holding presence and awareness with myself and a thousand-plus-pound being while remembering to breathe.

At the end of our session, I got on top of Cody. I wrapped my legs around his belly, leaned back, and rested my head on the base of his back right above his hips. I gazed into the vast blue sky and felt the stability and strength of his body as his hooves grounded into the earth.

For the first time in days, I let go. I breathed — inhale and exhale — surrendered, and leaned into the support. I felt at home and held and knew I was in a safe place to be honest, vulnerable, and brave.

At the close of our time together, Rachel took one look at me and proclaimed, "Something tells me this is exactly the healing medicine you need."

We heal in the presence of horses. We learn to experience and process emotions as they do. Horses are sensitive and have the capacity to feel another's feelings and hold a neutral, compassionate space. Interacting with these animals can be immensely therapeutic physically, mentally, and spiritually. They help to reawaken our potential to heal imbalances in our modern-day lives.

Rachel and Cody awakened something in me. Something I didn't forecast or know how to bring to life. For years I bargained with my restlessness and substituted it with different things. When my hands touched Cody, I felt alive. Cody ignited my internal flame and brought me out of the overcast light and into the sunshine of my soul. Everything and everyone would brighten and illuminate — my world got sweeter and life felt complete.

Showing up without your mask, letting your guard down, and expressing your emotions and deepest desires is both beautiful and scary and not for the faint of heart. It is a practice of getting out of our way, breaking down and through old habits that hold us back, and ultimately learning to trust our inspiration and ourselves. It is in the moments of discomfort that we stretch our comfort zone and experience the extraordinary.

The Universe aligns in ways not always in agreement with our preferences, rules, or how we think things should go but instead with what we need.

Practice

Try this meditative practice.

Take five to ten minutes and find a quiet space. Sit or lie down in a comfortable, supported position. Use pillows or blankets to support you. Set your intention by inviting the body, mind, and heart to rest. First, notice your breath as it is in its natural state. Then, when you feel ready, begin to guide the breath and take a few deep breaths in and out through your nose, ensuring the breath is smooth and even in length, perhaps working up to a four-count inhale followed by a four-count exhale. If comfortable, you can work toward an exhale that is twice as long as your inhale. For example, inhale at a four-count and exhale at an eight-count. When you feel complete, let the breath rest and hold awareness with your body.

Slow down your attention, rest in the stillness, and practice silent listening. Set the orientation to an open, sincere, and curious mindset, as if not knowing but ready to discover something and allow space and time for understanding to arise in its natural timing without a sense of urgency.

Find out if there is any guidance or inspiration, any suggestions from your soul. It can be quite subtle.

If yes, take note, remember, and plan to move forward with this information. It may be a word, color, sensation, insight. If nothing comes, trust that you have all the guidance you need right now. There is no right or wrong way to do this.

When we learn to rest our minds we have the ability to hear our soul.

There are many faces and names for ways inspiration can manifest, i.e., intuition, gut instinct, heart knowing, etc. It arises in the gut and heart and touches a deep and emotional place within. Like a superpower, when it strikes, its nature is so powerful that it asks of you something greater than yourself and gives you the energy to act. There may be initial hesitation, but the nudge, the voice inside, says to do it anyway. It may not always align with your expectations and plans; however, it is the truest offering of you.

Writing Prompts

How do you honor inspiration?

_____

_____

_____

_____

_____

_____

_____

_____

_____

_____

_____

_____

_____

_____

_____

_____

_____

_____

What happened when you answered the call of inspiration?
How did it feel, what was the outcome?

_____

_____

_____

_____

_____

_____

_____

_____

_____

_____

_____

_____

_____

_____

_____

_____

_____

_____

_____

_____

What happened when you didn't answer the call?
How did it feel, what was the outcome?

_____

_____

_____

_____

_____

_____

_____

_____

_____

_____

_____

_____

_____

_____

_____

_____

_____

_____

_____

_____

CHAPTER 2

The Afterglow of the Unknown

"The process of moving from what we don't know
to what we are to learn is a process that can be trusted.
It's how we grow and change. It's okay to not know.
It's okay to let ourselves move into knowing.
The lesson is trusting that we'll know when it's time."

MELODY BEATTIE

December 26, 2021 continued. It was my first session, and I was amazed at how good it felt to groom a horse. I had no idea of the limitless benefits of this simple act.

Though first intimidated by Cody's size, I felt the warmth of his body move up my arm and into my chest. My breath elongated and smoothed, inviting any last tension to melt.

In the relaxation process, horses release oxytocin — a bonding hormone and powerful neurotransmitter released from the brain and horse. It helps regulate human-to-human and human-to-animal relationships. The increase in oxytocin levels results in more rewarding relationships and increased levels of fulfillment, peace, and joy.

Meeting Cody was as if meeting a much-anticipated crush for the first time. I had experienced the glow and was mesmerized by the mystery of horses and their intuitive healing abilities. An energy inhabited that day and the coming months, almost like a second heart beating in my chest.

I understood the "horse high" and the addictive hold it would have over me after our first encounter. Initially intending to be a few sessions with Cody and Rachel, it turned into a five-month adventure and weekly road trips up to the ranch.

As I explored uncharted territory, my stability was my courage and faith. My curiosity, presence, desire to play, readiness to push my edge of comfort and skillset, and undoubtedly, Cody and Rachel were the conditions that induced this euphoric feeling and would hold me steady and accountable over the next five months.

It can be tempting to stay home or bypass something new out of fear of failure or the unknown. Stepping out of our comfort zone is a practice of effort and discipline. When we practice being comfortable with discomfort, we stretch our capacity and build the belief that we can do the unfamiliar, even when it is both daunting and beautiful.

The excitement of trying something new has not always come with ease. The paralyzing fear and restrictions I placed on myself and that once held me hostage dissolves as I shed layers of conditioned beliefs. When I witness the exhilaration and benefits of my efforts, I recognize my infinite potential.

In the presence of Cody, I was able to choreograph a confident result in the face of uncertainty, resulting in feelings of strength, capability, and pleasure. Rather than my habitual relationship around uncertainty that I once associated with danger or "flight-or-fight." Through the lens of inspiration and curiosity versus fear and judgment, I created a new pathway, revealing that uncertainty can sometimes lead to delight and fulfillment.

Immediately and after our time together, I felt an increased sense of creativity and intuition. I would soon discover this feeling would linger, grow, and expand the more I exercised my faith in the mystery.

At some point on our spiritual journey, we are required to take a leap of faith into the unknown. To step outside our familiar context, embrace what we do not know, and trust the unforeseen vistas as they open along our path and broaden our horizons.

Practice

Prompting Play: A mindfulness practice and invitation to play.

Begin by making a list. Include activities and things of interest, things you dream about doing, things that excite and scare you, and the many ways you played as a child. The act of creating a list will help inspire and motivate your memory, intuition, creativity, and desire to play and experiment. Choose one of the activities on your list. Commit and set an intention to play at least once during your day for seven days. Set aside time for play, like you would a necessary appointment. It could be for five minutes or five hours. Start with what is realistic and watch how the essence of space and play expands and unfolds into your days and weeks.

Writing Prompts

What is something you want to try,
but the fear of the unknown or failure holds you back?

_____

_____

_____

_____

_____

_____

_____

_____

_____

_____

_____

_____

_____

_____

_____

_____

_____

_____

Reflect on a time when you took a leap of faith and braved your heart. What did you discover and how did it influence your journey? Describe your experience in detail with sensations and vivid narrative.

CHAPTER 3

Learning to Ride

*"Such moments of communion between you and
the living earth can open doorways into a more magical,
mysterious, and meaningful life."*

MICAH MORTALI

January 1, 2021. The first day I rode Cody. The landscape was a geography of possibility, and the air fresh and invigorating. Sporting my navy down jacket and borrowed rider's helmet, I was warmhearted and ready. The sky was opaque and ashen with a striking thin misty layer of shadowy silver patches of clouds, stretching and spanning as far as the eyes could see. Sheer enough for the buttery light of the sun to illuminate a soft, creamy blemish in the wild blue. The threadlike rays of the sun kissed my cheeks and were a warm invitation to soften any lingering reservations.

Against the backdrop of the sky, Cody and I were one, a silhouette to be seen, a grin stretching as expansive as the sky. Rachel wanted to try me bareback, with no stirrups or saddle to secure and to test my sense of balance and security on the back of Cody. With nothing but a thin pad and layer of cushion between our bodies, I felt the strength of his bones as I settled my pelvis firmly on the ridge of his back, my torso lengthening delicately over my sit bones.

I got acquainted with the skills of riding. I learned how to get Cody to walk and stay on the ring dirt trail outlined in the dewy green grass. I learned how to stop and ask Cody to hoe and to turn around and go the opposite direction.

Rachel taught me to execute clarity around my intention with resolve and focus. To visualize the direction and desired outcome before requesting Cody. She coached me on posture and placement of my body — head, neck, shoulders, spine, torso, chest, arms, hands, legs, and feet. She familiarized me with the subtleties of the reins and leg pressure, when to release and pull back, when to apply, and when to back off. She taught me how to use vocal commands and when to infuse them to obtain my desired outcome. Not to mention the constant cues to come back to my body and breathe. First and foremost, Rachel prompted me to stay present and aware, calm but keenly alert, head and gaze forward, and eye on the prize.

Cody tested me moment by moment. If I did not stay in tune with his and my body and energy, he would lose interest and slow his pace. In the split second I got caught up in my thoughts and attention went adrift or exhibited signs of nervousness or frustration, Cody would sense the confusion and doubt and veer off course or stop.

Through the many layers, skills, and multisensory aspects of learning to ride a horse, I was learning to connect with my internal instincts. To be assertive but not aggressive, authentic and clear with my request, to work in partnership, and when to take the lead and command respect.

As the rider, I needed to mirror the horse's qualities — his openness, sensitivity, adaptability, and observance — to harmonize and work in collaboration. My focus and balance, stillness amid activity, restful approach to learning and developing a new skill-set, and capacity to complement Cody's natural abilities created the desirable conditions for an inspiring display of human-horse connection.

Practice

Create a daily intention ritual.

Take one or more minutes in the morning (before you check your phone, messages, emails, or work, etc.) to pause and start your day with intention. Keep a daily intention journal and write down a word or more. Stay attentive and watch how your day unfolds. Commit to doing this for seven days or longer. Reflect at the end of the day or week, did your day flow, and align with more intention and awareness? The shifts in our day can often be tiny and subtle. Stay keenly aware and be open to discovery.

Writing Prompts

Write about a time when presence, focus, will, and an open, curious mindset created the desirable conditions for connection.

_____

_____

_____

_____

_____

_____

_____

_____

_____

_____

_____

_____

_____

_____

_____

_____

_____

_____

_____

Where in your life can you foster a restful approach to learning when challenged with developing a new skillset?

_____

_____

_____

_____

_____

_____

_____

_____

_____

_____

_____

_____

_____

_____

_____

_____

_____

_____

_____

_____

CHAPTER 4

Practicing Presence

*"...When we learn how to relax into the present moment,
we learn how to relax with the unknown."*

PEMA CHÖDRÖN

There is something about being with a horse that offers a powerful invitation to slow down, breathe, become present, and connect with an open and curious mind and heart. One of the most powerful life lessons that horses offer us is that everything begins with exploring the relationship with ourselves.

Horses allow us to turn our attention inward and genuinely restore connection and compassion with ourselves and our innate wisdom. This permission to discover the subtleties of our own emotions, needs, and desires shows us that we truly need, in any moment, to feel safe enough to let go and hold a gentle presence with what is and show up as our authentic selves.

January 17, 2021. My fourth visit to the ranch. Rachel mentioned she wanted to facilitate a meditation with Finn and me. Up until this point, I was building a relationship with Cody.

Without too much overthinking and hesitation, I found myself sitting in an expandable camping chair and holding the lead rope that was attached to Finn's halter. There he was, this thousand-plus-pound being standing before me in all his beauty and magnificence. It was both intimidating and exhilarating. I was scared shitless.

As I fidgeted in my chair and laughed nervously, Finn flirted. He gently nuzzled the tip of his nose and mouth on my shoulders, kissed my forehead, nibbled at my hair, and poked at my thighs and feet. I was tight, tense, and guarded. My heart raced, my palms were clammy, my mind began to spin, and my breath was shallow — worry was written all over my face.

Rachel curiously asked, "What are you afraid of?" "I am afraid he is going to bite me," I said. "He is not going to bite you," she replied. I was a bit relieved but not entirely. After all, I only met Rachel a couple of months ago. We were still building trust, and I was building confidence in horses. I was building trust and confidence in myself.

Then, something shifted. Once I declared my fear out loud, it no longer had a powerful hold. The fidgeting stopped, my breath deepened, and I closed my eyes. I connected to my core and the earth below. Like a mantra, I repeated silently, "You will be OK, you will be OK."

My breath was my friendly companion and doorway into the moment and my heart.

I leaned into my vulnerability and discomfort and embraced my fear. I began to relax and my energy shifted to one of curiosity and fearlessness.

I tasted the residue from my tears. I felt the sun touching my skin and Finn's breath on my cheek as our inhales and exhales began to sync. With my bodily senses immersed, my experience heightened, and the feeling of presence enhanced. I was free to feel and let go. I accepted Finn's invitation to dance and hold space.

My body softened and stilled. I held an open and gentle presence with my emotions without turning away or distracting. I allowed the feelings to move through me without manipulation. I was purely being.

I watched as apprehension turned to tears, relief, and immense gratitude. A lightness lapped over me like the coolness of shade on a hot summer's day. Giddiness, joy, and laughter filled the air.

From a very young age, I associated fear and discomfort as an indicator that harm was near. My imagination ran wild, fantasizing worst-case scenarios. I did my best to avoid being uncomfortable. The avoidance became a habit, and the momentum of the habit carried and grew with time.

Learning to hold a gentle presence with my discomfort and to embrace my fears is a continual practice. Finn reminded me it is OK to be scared and reflected my ability to build trust, practice staying with emotions, and that it is safe to do so.

I undid something that day, something I was once tethered to. I surrendered to Finn, my experience, and something greater than us both.

When we practice within the realm of our daily lives and with the flow of our emotions, we nourish the art of staying versus running away. We generate curiosity, courage, and stability. We begin the groundwork for a calm, clear, strong mind.

Practice

Commit to practicing presence for one minute or more a day for seven days or more. Get out of the narrative of your mind and into the moment. Take a relaxed approach and practice being with things as they change without manipulation, judgement, or expectation. Avoid doing anything and simply allow yourself to show up and just be. Catch on to moments of discomfort and hold a gentle presence and compassionate space for the sensations that arise within.

Writing Prompt

What does it mean to embrace the totality of your experience and hold a gentle presence with what is?

_____

_____

_____

_____

_____

_____

_____

_____

_____

_____

_____

_____

_____

_____

_____

_____

_____

Write about a time you embraced fear.
What emotions and sensations came up for you?
What was the outcome of that experience?

_____

_____

_____

_____

_____

_____

_____

_____

_____

_____

_____

_____

_____

_____

_____

_____

_____

_____

_____

_____

CHAPTER 5

Potential and Possibility

*"Put your heart, mind, and soul into even your smallest acts.
This is the secret of success."*

SWAMI SIVANANDA

February 6, 2021. The empty sky was an absolute blue, the air crisp and clean. Another day at the ranch full of potential and possibility.

Upon arrival after our usual tea and chat, Rachel invited me to go into the pasture alone and get Cody for our lesson.

Hesitant and eager, I grabbed the halter and lead rope. With optimism, I walked toward the open pasture. I opened the gate and paused to catch my breath. The warmth of the sun thawing the layers of resistance. The whisper of the wind gentle against my body and the smell of sweet grass and wet dirt beneath my boots familiar. I set my intention — to be open, curious, playful, present, confident, and connected.

I turned the corner to meet myself in the mirror. Cody was grazing and nibbling at the grass. My heart pulsated, and I was overcome with delight as the sensation of butterflies burned in my belly. I stood a couple of feet away, bribing him with the tender call of my voice, requesting his attention with no avail. I walked closer and rubbed his shoulder and withers. Cool, calm, and carefree, Cody was undisturbed by my presence.

After twenty minutes, Rachel texted to ask if everything was OK. I replied, "It's going OK, but I have one little problem. How do I distract him from the grass and get his head up?"

To get his attention, she said I could poke at his nose or place the lead rope around his neck and gently pull. With my fear of being bit, the first option was unappealing. So, I put the rope around his neck and gave a little tug — not wanting to hurt him, yet not forceful enough with my intent. Cody did not budge.

Secretively stubborn and wise, Cody was putting me to the test. He was patient, unlike me. I felt a tiny tantrum building up. I felt defeated but sure I wanted to do this on my own.

Another ten minutes went by before I texted Rachel again. This time I told her to come in ten minutes if I did not come out of the pasture with Cody. I was even more determined and willing. She believed in me. It was time to trust and believe in myself. I took a deep breath, set a clear intention, and tugged with more assertion on the lead rope.

After a while, curiosity got the better of Cody and he lifted his gaze and followed my lead. Still a little unsure but getting braver by the minute, I cautiously led him toward the direction of the gate.

We arrived at the bare dusty dirt patch just before the white fence and gate. Void of any appetizing grass to tempt his attention, we paused and had a moment of celebration. Overcome with gratitude and love, tears of joy glistened my eyes. I hugged him, and I let him nuzzle me with his nose and face.

I secured the halter around his face and, with a wide-eyed grin, proceeded through the gate lead rope in hand with Cody close behind.

I experienced another breakthrough and proud moment on this journey back to my wild heart.

The familiar feelings of timidness and frustration arose when Cody ignored my gentle gestures. I began to doubt my leadership abilities and horsemanship capabilities. Cody was consistent, willing, quiet, and responsive in my effort for his interest once I exerted my assertiveness and assurance, a way to provide me with my dignity while accomplishing the goal.

When we persist with open and earnest effort coupled with curiosity, courage, consistency, and will, we break through old habits and conditions, expanding into our infinite potential. We shed outdated limitations and stories that hold us back for fear of failure, rejection, or disbelief.

Cody mirrored the cowgirl in me who desires sincere and subtle grace, confidence, and freedom to be who I am. The one that tastes fear but is now brave enough to push the edge of discomfort.

Often in life, it isn't the big things that happen to us that have the most profound effect; it's the little things.

Practice

When we aspire to become sincere, curious, and consistent in our efforts, we discover the will and capability to break through old habits and conditions. Take some time to reflect on a habit or mental condition that you want to change or remove. This could be a negative thought pattern that you repeat or a daily habit such as mindlessly scrolling through social media. Make a list of one or more habits or conditions you want to change. When ready, pick one that feels doable and easy, something you can implement each day with consistency and accountability.

A couple examples might include: Making a vow to take a social media detox or maybe it's a negative thought pattern or belief that is no longer serving you that you want to change, i.e., thoughts of doubt that appear in moments of frustration or when trying something new. Simply catch on to when they arise and take a moment to pause and take a few conscious breaths, interrupting the pattern.

Make a commitment to do this daily for seven days or more. Set yourself up for accountability. How will you remind yourself to do this every day? Keep a small notebook or track on your phone or a piece of paper to help remind you and track your progress. Experiment and see what works for you to help you remember your practice.

Writing Prompts

Reflect on the little things in your life that have
had the most profound effect.

_____

_____

_____

_____

_____

_____

_____

_____

_____

_____

_____

_____

_____

_____

_____

_____

_____

_____

_____

_____

_____

How did you feel when you worked through familiar
messages of doubt and persisted with courage and consistency
to achieve your desired outcome?

_____

_____

_____

_____

_____

_____

_____

_____

_____

_____

_____

_____

_____

_____

_____

_____

_____

_____

_____

CHAPTER 6

Practice Makes Progress (Not Perfect)

"Everything that lives needs space to grow and to become."

THICH NHAT HANH

It had been over a month since Rachel and I started working together. We had been rehearsing and refining my skillset each time I stepped foot into the outdoor arena. I was acquiring the art and craft of a smooth and transparent transition between a stop, walk and trot, and maintaining a trot for a total length of the ring.

Each session, we were building and layering upon knowledge and skills — how to be alert of my surroundings, safety, presence, breath, recognizing body language and energy, purpose, the power of focus and visualization, and less on loud vocal commands or instruction.

I aspired to reach my desired result effortlessly, whether walking or trotting or working on seamless transitions without harboring the usual expectations of trying to get it right or perfect.

The minute you relax your effort and connection is the moment the horse will perceive the situation differently, thinking you want something other than what you are aspiring toward and slow down, veer off course, or stop. The rider must stay active and in constant communication with the horse.

A proper relationship between horse and rider is an act of true teamwork, leadership, and respect. An active rider must notice the subtleties of energy and pressure with every gesture while maintaining attention and clear direction to ignite and sustain connection, ease, and flow.

After a few weeks, I noticed our sessions were triggering and bringing up a lot of unresolved trauma around doubt, fear, lack of confidence, patterns of the inner critic, disapproval, and embarrassment — the habit of wanting to be perfect. I scripted fictional stories and assumed Rachel was judging me because I was not "getting it" fast enough. I caught on to the repetitive narrative, judgment, and familiar stories that I was a slow learner and not good enough.

When I panicked or got caught up in my head, doubting my innate abilities, my body would brace and tense. I gripped the reins, pulled back, and held my breath — unintentionally, energetically blocking Cody and disrupting the flow of connection.

Horses bring themselves, with no thoughts of doubt, am I doing this right, or do they like me. They hold pure presence and meet you at a place of neutrality. They know when you are unsure and inauthentic.

When I leaned into discomfort and trusted my capacity, our capabilities together, and allowed myself to be perfectly imperfect, this prompted the release of worries and doubts.

This lesson would come up repeatedly for many weeks, but that is the beauty of showing up, being consistent, and holding yourself accountable.

Cody's reflection portrayed the more sensitive, empathetic, creative, intuitive, and confident person I was becoming. He reminded me to hold presence over perfection, honor my pace, and remove any false or artificial timelines around my process. A foundation and relationship built on trust and at a pace that allowed us both to feel safe and held.

Practice

Getting good at celebrating.

Make a list of habits, activities, or behaviors you currently do and a list of practices, actions, or behaviors you want to establish. For instance, one could be creating a daily habit of flossing your teeth, drinking more water, going for a walk, showing up, or remembering your spiritual or self-care practices. Explore and get creative. There are no limitations.

Choose one item on the list, start easy and small. Each time you do the daily activity or thing, immediately celebrate that you did it and remembered to do it. Hold a feeling of gratitude. Delight in your celebration by adding an emotionally positive and sincere feeling to your celebration.

Your celebration is unique to you. It could be repeating "good job" out loud or internally to yourself or singing and dancing to your favorite song or smiling or placing your hands to your heart as a gesture of devotional recognition. There is no right or wrong way to do this — experiment with what works for you.

How will you remember to celebrate? You might try writing it down on a Post-it or reminder on your phone. Again, experiment here and see what sticks.

What if you do the good deed or act but forget to celebrate immediately after, only to remember later? Not to worry, celebrate when you remember to celebrate!

By celebrating the good act with an emotional charge, we build energy and momentum around the act. The more you do it, the faster it will get wired into the brain as a habit with a positive association. The heart and core of celebration is the feeling. Each time you remember to celebrate the good deed, it will integrate, grow, and expand. The more capable you will be able to tap into the spontaneity of celebration with time and practice.

Writing Prompts

What does it mean to you to trust your process
and honor your pace?

_____

_____

_____

_____

_____

_____

_____

_____

_____

_____

_____

_____

_____

_____

_____

_____

_____

_____

How often do you override your pace and why?

_____

_____

_____

_____

_____

_____

_____

_____

_____

_____

_____

_____

_____

_____

_____

_____

_____

_____

_____

_____

CHAPTER 7

Feeling Alive

"After excitement we are so restful.
When the thumb of fear lifts, we are so alive."

MARY OLIVER

Sometimes in those unplanned and unexpected moments is when you feel most alive.

March 26, 2021. It was just like every other Saturday. I was on Cody rehearsing my riding skills in the arena and Rachel was next to us doing groundwork with Selena, her 3-year-old wild mustang. After some minor instruction, Rachel left me alone to explore my transitions from walk to trot and back to walk and stop. With the removal of the self-imposed pressures I would undergo from being watched and fewer distractions and reminders from Rachel, I was less in my thoughts and more in rhythm with my body and Cody.

I was calm, quiet, and receptive enough to feel his presence and my own, sensitive and adaptable enough to follow its guidance, and spontaneous enough to move with its flow. We were in similar frequency.

Cody and I were riding in a comfortable trot when Rachel vocally prompted Selena into a canter. Cody, taking the cue, unexpectedly changed speeds and loped into a canter. I was flying on air, feeling the sensory union between strength and gentleness of grace and movement beneath my body. As soon as I realized what was happening, Cody's speed slowed and stopped. Startled and thrilled, a tidal wave of repressed emotion washed over my body. Salty teardrops of joy glistened and fell from my eyes as I laughed in amazement. I couldn't quite believe what had just happened. I had been curious about cantering, but it was not a transition and skill I was formally taught.

The "rider's high." A rush of confidence, composure, and clarity unleashed when one's control of a thousand-pound being begins to flow like a flash of hope rising.

As humans, we are encouraged to deny the body's wisdom and dissociate from instincts and senses. Over time, I adopted fearful and restrictive habits that inhibited my freedom of movement and authentic expression of who I am.

The treasures of riding are physical, emotional, and spiritual. Horses teach us how to have flexible boundaries, emotional congruence, creative visualization, and clarity of intent. When you align yourself with the flow of nature's currents, you truly make that connection with the horse.

There is a spot inside a horse, an opening where there is no fear or resistance. The same sweet spot I was uncovering and opening within myself.

The most exciting moments happened when I liberated my physical and emotional concerns through Cody's mirroring. Remembering to sit steady and buoyant, lengthen through my spine, soften my shoulders, relax my arms and grip, unclench my jaw, breathe deep while holding presence, attention, and focus. I was learning to master a complex array of skills while rekindling a relationship with myself through the horse, with collaboration and sensitivity rather than fear and intimidation.

Riding a horse feels like a series of small surprises and revelations rewarded by surges of pleasure. It is a feeling of music in motion, of sublime silence between two souls. It is beyond the words of description.

To understand a horse and have willing communication, you must develop awareness and discipline within yourself. All the ground-work Cody and I did together — consistency, commitment, and dedication — led me to this moment. The more present and aware, the less scared I was and apt to concoct "what if" scenarios of all the things that could go bad. I was learning how to become a more confident rider, a more humble and secure woman.

Each breakthrough building upon one another, an invitation to let go, and deeper exploration into the mystery and expansion of my soul. The different gaits of a horse began to represent the different gateways into my heart.

With consistent, committed, dedicated, and devotional practice and self-study, we develop awareness, accountability, and discipline. When we hold presence and learn to relax into and trust the body and inner wisdom, life unexpectedly opens, expands, and naturally flows in harmony with universal flow, like a river to a lake, a stream to an ocean.

Practice

A daily practice to see through a beginner's mind and eyes.

Recall what it was like to walk into a new relationship, activity, class, job, experience, or event, to begin something new without any prior knowledge or expectation. Call forth this memory and begin your day with the intention to see through beginner's eyes, through the eyes of innocence. Create an aspiration to walk into a new or familiar experience with an open, curious, willing, present, and playful mindset. Do this for seven days or more. Use the journal pages in this book to keep track of what comes up for you. Notice what kind of mindset allows for that innocent, curious flow and what kind of mindset disrupts the flow of innocence.

Writing Prompts

Reflect on one or more moments in your life when you felt most alive. Were the experiences unplanned or unexpected? Describe in detail with as much description as you can remember.

_____

_____

_____

_____

_____

_____

_____

_____

_____

_____

_____

_____

_____

_____

_____

_____

_____

_____

_____

_____

_____

What were the qualities and conditions that created this feeling?

CHAPTER 8

Compassionate Connection

"Only the development of compassion and understanding for others can bring us the tranquility and happiness we all seek."

DALAI LAMA

April. I woke one Saturday morning feeling a subtle sense of sorrow and impatience. There was not one or more reasons triggering my mood. It just was, though my mind was searching for answers. The feelings lingered on my drive up to the ranch. My energy and enthusiasm were low, but my spirit was reaching and guiding me in the direction I needed to go that morning.

When I walked into the pasture and met Cody's body, tears glistened my parched eyes and throat. There was no holding back. Each droplet was an invitation to soften my subtle tight jaw and release the gripping and tension in my neck and shoulders that I had been holding — to be vulnerable and express myself.

What were the ingredients to this recipe of release and subtle sacred connection? Was it the generous, open, and grounded heart of Cody? Was it my open, willing, courageous heart in an endless search for connection and liberation? Could it have been the stable earth beneath my feet, expansive land, vast sky above, and warm sun kissing my skin?

It was all that and more.

At the forefront of my chest and throat was sadness that stemmed from the world's weight, endings, new beginnings, and a longing to be heard and seen — to feel a sense of connection and belonging.

If my voice could speak, what would it say? What was my body holding?

When our eyes met, I gazed into the soul of Cody, and I knew there was no hiding. I had two choices; I could fake it and stay reserved or speak sincerely from my heart. I chose the latter.

My words trembled with inhibition. At first glance, shying away. A habit long ago created to protect my innocent spirit. I spoke even with trepidation because, for me, there is no other choice but to practice being my most authentic self. Cody set the conditions. Held in his warm embrace, it was safe to be me without repercussions.

I've always felt connected to horses. They invite me to tune in to a part of myself that seems more ancient, mysterious, beautiful, and intuitive, as if I have resurrected a lost part of myself.

I believe it's because horses embody true presence and authenticity.

Unlike humans, horses hold no personal belief structures, thoughts of the past or worries of the future, no self-doubt or judgment, just the pureness of presence. They meet you in a place of neutrality.

Horses allow us to turn our attention inward to genuinely restore connection with ourselves and our innate wisdom. This permission to discover the subtleties of our own emotions, needs, and desires shows us what we truly need — in any moment — to feel safe enough to be utterly ourselves.

When we are in connection with self and others, love and energy flow, and we feel a deep sense of presence, purpose, and meaning. There is a willingness and open opportunity to be heard and seen and to see another deeply. To learn and understand something about ourselves and the other. Below the layers of fear, anger, resentment, close-mindedness, and confusion reside discomfort and sadness. Below that lies a longing to connect and belong.

We are highly social beings with a hardwired need for love, connection, and a true sense of belonging. The more connected we feel, the better choices we make energetically, and our life ripens with gratitude and compassion, dissolving the illusion that separates us from ourselves, one another, all of Mother Earth.

Practice

Recognize moments of connection throughout your day. Linger longer when you do and notice how you feel. You can do this practice with the smallest thing or moment. Do this with people you know, with strangers, with people that challenge you or that you dislike, with yourself, your partner, children, fur babies, etc. The possibilities are endless. Start easy and work your way toward the more challenging people or moments.

Writing Prompts

What qualities signify deep connection?

_____

_____

_____

_____

_____

_____

_____

_____

_____

_____

_____

_____

_____

_____

_____

_____

_____

_____

How do you recognize connection?

_____

_____

_____

_____

_____

_____

_____

_____

_____

_____

_____

_____

_____

_____

_____

_____

_____

_____

_____

_____

_____

What gets in the way of connection?

_____

_____

_____

_____

_____

_____

_____

_____

_____

_____

_____

_____

_____

_____

_____

_____

_____

_____

_____

_____

CHAPTER 9

Awakening

"Don't hesitate if you unexpectedly feel joy — give into it...
It could be anything, but very likely you notice it in the instant
when love begins."

MARY OLIVER

May. The time is growing close when I must say goodbye to Cody and Rachel as they venture to a new home and state. An agreement I knew and agreed to when I signed our soul contract in December. Cody, Rachel, and the gang are embedded in my DNA. We are kindred spirits and will always be a symbol in one another's lives.

For a long time, I watched my desire and felt an emptiness growing inside. Then the delight, when my inspiration signaled and my courage kindled and I stepped onto new ground, a path of unexpected plenitude opened before me. Though my destination was not clear, I trusted the promise of the opening as I unfurled myself into the grace of a new beginning.

I will miss my Saturday morning ritual of driving up to the ranch, my home away from home, as I hummed along to some of my favorite playlists and podcasts while drinking tea or coffee. I will miss the smells and sights of the country roads — the long stretch of yellow mustards, the thick trunks of the eucalyptus trees that extend like ornaments along Lakeville Highway, the shabby ghost barns, ranches, and grazing horses and livestock. I will miss the way the light hit the water at dusk, creating a baby blue and lavender mist along the horizon of Highway 37 as the sun set in the rearview mirror. I will miss idling in traffic, windows rolled down, as I listened to the call of the red-winged blackbird, body tired, heart full of satisfaction and gratitude for another long and beautiful Saturday, reminding me of the abundance in each moment.

On the other side of sorrow is joy and in between and all around is beauty, tenderness, and love — should you open your heart and eyes to believe and see. Sometimes we don't know what is missing until we try something new, stepping out of our comfort and into our hearts.

The spark of joy I felt with Cody was the moment when love began. Joy was the drug, and love was the hangover that kept me coming back for more.

I was afraid to ride a horse. When I met Cody, my fear was big but my courage was bigger. We had an honor code. He taught me how to ride a horse with confidence, become a leader, and hold space. He reminded me of my capacity to step out of the mold I so carefully created and show up, mutating my fear into grace.

A horse understands the secret to life. They flow with presence and are regal and exquisite, wild and playful. In those moments when we would canter around the ring, flashes of clarity mixed with waves of delight flowed as a stream of automatic response. An incredible wave of ecstasy filled my body, resurrecting lost parts of myself.

To give into joy is to give into love. It is to give into life. It is consent to live outside the confines of our past, without expectation or a grand master plan. To experience joy is to see life through a new lens and witness beauty without distraction. A blessing to step away from our day-to-day and expose ourselves to discover joy in unforeseen places, nooks, and crannies.

Walking this path with Cody opened vistas in my interior landscape that were previously concealed from view. I learned how to let my guard down long enough to learn how to trust. Cody showed me how to embrace my imperfections and habits, encouraging me to become more natural and authentic with myself and with him and to greater humility and empathy toward my journey and that of another.

To find unexpected joy and give into it will change your life. It will illuminate your heart, so the branches of love extend to things you never thought or planned. To fall in love with another being reflects our inherent capacity to love, to experience joy.

I am learning to love what is mortal, to hold it against my bones, and when the time comes to let it go, to let it go. I am learning that we can hold grief and joy simultaneously and that emotion is not black or white but a beautiful blend of living and expressing ourselves authentically while embracing the vastness of our human experience.

It is a bittersweet goodbye — a close of a chapter and a mysterious beginning of another yet again. I never knew I needed Rachel until she found me. I never knew I needed Cody until he unearthed me. Joy was what I needed to fall in love with life again. It was the balm to my spirit and medicine to my soul.

Cody liberated the untamed woman, the cowgirl, and awakened the intimacy of a horse within.

My prayer and invitation to you is to live without holding back, learn to find ease in risk, trust in the leap, and surrender to the soar. To awaken your spirit to adventure and come home to a new rhythm. Listen for the call, take the dive. Your soul senses the world that awaits you. Life is worth living, and you are worth it.

Practice

Recognizing Joy: A mindfulness practice for every day.

We all have the capacity to feel joy, yet happiness and joy can feel elusive. It often gets shrouded in moments of distraction by our preconceived conditions, habitual ways of living, and thoughts. Joy as a recognition practice can open our eyes to the inherent joy and beauty within and how our external world can reflect that capacity within. The more we recognize and water happiness and joy, the more it will become second nature and like a seed, will grow and thrive.

When we can aspire to see the joy in ourselves, in others, in nature, in the moment, our world expands, blooms, and brightens. We awaken to sacred connection leaving little room for the coloring of condition, judgment, or opinion. It is the doorway to accepting what is and witnessing the elusive joy we misplace when caught up in the past or future.

Set an intention each day to notice joy. Be open, willing, and curious. Recognize moments of happiness and joy, hold a whole-hearted presence with your experience, no matter how long or brief. Allow yourself to linger longer in those moments. See what happens. Do you notice any shifts within you? What was the moment that brought forth this sense of joy? What inhibits joy? Use the pages in this book to reflect and take notes.

Remain open to the moment and be willing to experience the joy that is always there.

Writing Prompts

Write what it means to you to love what is mortal,
to hold it against your bones, and when the time comes
to let it go, to let it go.

_____

_____

_____

_____

_____

_____

_____

_____

_____

_____

_____

_____

_____

_____

_____

_____

_____

_____

Write of a time when the end of one chapter opened to
a beautiful, unexpected beginning.

_____

_____

_____

_____

_____

_____

_____

_____

_____

_____

_____

_____

_____

_____

_____

_____

_____

_____

_____

_____

_____

CHAPTER 10

Poetry of Spirit

*"It is only by slowing down that we can hear the spirit
whisper inside. It is only in the depths of stillness that we detect
the prescient of something vast and subtle, something
inexhaustible and immense, a pervasive force
much greater than our own small self.*

TIAS LITTLE

A Cibecue Apache Elder once said, "The purpose of sacred land is to protect the place and to perfect the human mind. Wisdom sits in places."

Whatever you don't know, the land and horses will teach you. Land instructs us, so do horses. So do miles of yellow mustard country roads. So does the soft stillness of the morning. So does the call of the red-winged blackbird as her melody carries in the wind. So does the single-file march of cows heading home at dusk. So does the flush of the horizon as the sunset brushes her masterpiece in the sky.

But we must be willing to listen and see the boundless teachings and messages bestowed before us.

The spirit of the ranch, the earth, and the drumming of hooves were instruments orchestrating music that only I could hear — a place of unwritten magic that swept across the land and etched my soul.

The energy and ambiance of the ranch were sacred, expansive, and plentiful in potential and collaboration. This place, Rachel, and her passionate and generous heart, meticulous and vast in wisdom and knowledge, Cody as mischievous as he was forgiving and dependable, had chosen me. Or had I chosen them? Or had we chosen at all?

The land and horses' wordless qualities took on a cleansing quality of space resting at the heart of the matter, redefining and disbanding my ideas around intelligence and intuition, pain and pleasure, curiosity and compassion, joy and sorrow, love and life.

Everything in nature invites us to be what we are. Horses hold us to what is present, to who we are in that moment and not who we've been, where we are headed, or how our "success" culturally defines us. What is evident to a horse is not the exaggeration of what we have accomplished or what material prizes we possess, but the root and core of truth and what is real within us: fear, anger, frustration, insecurity, compassion, sincerity, peace, and joy. We are transparent to them and thus vulnerable and exposed, a place where we can be ourselves.

A horse can uncover authenticity and set the stage for the truth to liberate you. Cody and I traveled to a forbidden land. He taught me the art of conceiving an essential connection between two beings. As we moved in harmony with one another, bringing me to a place of stillness and inward tranquility amid action. We somehow knew to rehearse and hum the poetry of each other's spirit.

Creating a relationship and the heart of the ride preserves an expansive, nurturing, and challenging quality, a balance between intellect and instinct, strength and grace, lightness and substance, holding on and letting go, spirituality and sensory.

My willingness to relinquish and untangle traditional ways of thinking and conditional beliefs and respond authentically strengthened
my ability to navigate through the unknown. To become more fluid
and adaptable, to embrace all experiences and emotions as meaningful information. These were some of the most valuable skills I
learned from Cody and continue to learn from horses.

I used to be impatient with life. I was always searching and pining
for purpose, meaning, and joy. Such restlessness has left me, and
even in those moments when life feels dull and uncertain, I know
I have the capacity to feel happiness and contentment, a source
within that will never diminish. Our experiences reflect what is
inherent and illuminate our ability to feel joy.

We never know what will be revealed or discovered when we follow
our heart and intuition and the call of inspiration. In this case, it
cracked me wide open, exposing old wounds, connecting me to
repressed passion I was once unsure how to access.

When the mind is calm and responsive, without effort, inspiration,
insight, the right guidance will reveal and whisper directions to
our soul. It is our responsibility to listen and act with courage,
care, and attention.

It is never too late to learn and try something new and embark on
a soul mission. It is a practice one can aspire to while acknowl-
edging and honoring one's pace and process. It is coming back
to this place even if you wander off and remembering how to call
your spirit back. It is a journey with no destination, an unending
process of undoing and becoming.

I placed no end, expectation, or agenda. I dove headfirst into this
journey, embracing each moment and riding as it came. I learned

to take hold of the reins and to relax, breathe through discomfort, and be open to the collaboration and mystery of existence.

Practice

Give your mind, body, and spirit rest. Take a mini or long retreat away from the day-to-day noise, constant stimulation, and forward motion of modern life, technology, work, parenting, errands, etc. Take a few moments or more each day in nature. Stand in place or go for a walk or hike in a safe and familiar place or perhaps even a new setting. Set an intention to notice the beauty and one or more things that give you a sense of wonder and awe. Maybe you see something new, and perhaps you notice something familiar with fresh eyes. Take in the sites and sounds that are both subtle and obvious. Be in no hurry or have no plan of expectation. Just allow yourself to be in the grace of Mother Earth. She is waiting to be seen, felt, and expressed. If possible and comfortable, take your shoes off. Feel your bare feet against the dirt or grass. Notice the ground beneath your feet, and imagine roots extending deep into the earth as you stand and breathe or walk.

If you cannot get outside, look outside your window and take a few conscious deep breaths. Breathe it all in, even if it is just the top of a tree, branch, or patch of sky. Notice how you feel.

Bring nature indoors. Open your window for the fresh air and sounds to come in. Add a houseplant or bouquet to the desk, table, or shelf. Find ways to bring the colors and vitality of the natural world inside.

Writing Prompts

Make a list of the things or events or humans or animals that call
your spirit back and awaken a sense of aliveness within.
Expand on one or more of the items. If you are unsure, reflect on
experiences in your life that have left an imprint, ones that made
you come alive and alert.

_____

_____

_____

_____

_____

_____

_____

_____

_____

_____

_____

_____

_____

_____

_____

_____

Write about a time when you dove headfirst into a new beginning or experience, one where you placed no expectation or agenda on the outcome. What did you learn? How did you feel?

_____

_____

_____

_____

_____

_____

_____

_____

_____

_____

_____

_____

_____

_____

_____

_____

_____

_____

_____

Acknowledgments

To my husband. You never expressed a moment of hesitation around my creative capabilities and ambitions. Because of you, I trusted and believed in myself, kept going, and followed my dreams no matter the outcome. Your support and belief in me, this journey, and this book have been a blessing and the encouragement I needed in those moments of doubt.

To my teacher Mynx Inatsugu who in January 2017 had me declare out loud my dream to become a published writer, whose wisdom and teachings have taught me how to activate my yoga, spiritual practice, and aspirations into daily hands-on practices and habits. Whose suggested practices, some of which I share and expand on in this book, continue to influence my everyday life and have a genuine impact on my sense of joy, peace, and fulfillment. The insight revealed continues to be the inspiration, courage, and backbone behind my growth and evolution.

To Jax. Always Jax. You are the best furry companion a girl could ask for. Your unconditional love, support, and belief in me opened my heart wide open and held me steady in an uncertain world. Thank you for reminding me to take breaks from writing and the screen with your gentle nudges to be held in my arms.

To the Get It Done team! Your support, encouragement, expertise, and professionalism over this past year and during the Tiny Book Course and the production of this book were the inspiration and accountability I needed to continue being brave and following my HUT! Reminding me each step of the way that I am good enough. That my book is good enough and that "success" is not in the outcome but the leap.

About the Author

Dina Varellas is a certified yoga teacher, writer, and facilitator of women's circles, who leads intuitive women's writing classes. She is the author of a personal blog and various publications and articles. Spiritual studies, daily practice, and Mother Nature balance and nurture her desire to teach, serve, and grow. Dina lives in Northern California, where she loves to spend time snuggling and dancing with her beloved cat, Jax, riding horses, and spending time with her husband adventuring.

Lightning Source UK Ltd.
Milton Keynes UK
UKHW021823301221
396406UK00006B/260